An important note: This book is not intended as a substitute for the medical recommendation of physicians or other health-care providers. Rather, it is intended to offer information to help the reader cooperate with physicians and health professionals in a mutual quest for optimum well-being. The content of this book that contains any medical information, supplement information, or references ("Medical Information") is for informational purposes only and does not constitute medical advice, nor is it intended to be a substitute for professional medical advice, diagnosis, or treatment. The Medical Information does not recommend or endorse any specific products, opinions, or other information that may be mentioned therein.

The publisher and the author are not responsible for any goods and/or services offered or referred to in this book and expressly disclaim all liability in connection with the fulfillment of orders for any such goods and/or services and for any damage, loss, or expense to person or property arising out of or relating to them. The author and the publisher assume no liability or responsibility for any errors or omissions in the content of any Medical Information. Reliance on any Medical Information is solely at your own risk.

Disclaimer: I am not a medical professional, naturopath, etc. This book is written for the purpose of sharing my personal experiences only. I am not offering medical advice, nor am I suggesting anyone take any of the supplements or medication I did. My experience may not be the same as others. Always speak with your doctor or healthcare professional before introducing any new supplement, medication, or exercise routine.

Table Of Contents

Introduction

If you're reading this book, then my heart goes out to you. Either yourself or one of your loved ones is coping with a difficult and perplexing health condition, known as Chronic Fatigue Syndrome (CFS), which is also known as   Myalgic Encephalomyelitis (ME).   From now on, I'll be referring to this disease simply as CFS.

In addition to dealing with the disorder itself, it can also be frustrating that it's not widely recognized in the medical community, and there is no confirmed diagnostic test for CFS. I'm sure you yourself can relate the countless doctors' visits and blood tests you've completed, with everything appearing normal.

Well-meaning friends may even suggest that perhaps this condition is in your head, or that you're suffering from depression. While well-intentioned, these can you feel even more discouraged.

I don't need to tell you that this illness has a fair share of deniers. It will rankle you. But I think that in general, as humans it's tough to really empathize with someone if you haven't experienced what they're going through. So, try to give your friends and loved ones some slack.

I chose to write about my experience because I know how it feels to suffer through this condition and not have any answers, or wonder if you're ever going to get better. I personally have experienced a huge improvement in my symptoms, to the point where my life has almost returned to 'normal', and I'm so grateful for that. However, everyone is different, and what worked for me may not work for you.

Despite how hopeless your situation seems to feel some days, there is light at the end of the tunnel! In his book "Always Looking Up: The Adventures of an Incurable Optimist", Michael J. Fox shared this piece of wisdom with us :

> *"Acceptance doesn't mean resignation; it means understanding that something is what it is and that there's got to be a way through it."*

That was true for the Parkinson's that Michael J. Fox is battling, and it is true for our fight with CFS.

Chapter One: H   ow I Developed CFS

Being active has always been my passion, and part of my identity. Some of my earliest childhood memories are of playing soccer with my dad, being on the track and field team, and going on long hikes. In my early thirties, I developed a passion for weightlifting. I took pride in my physique and my skill at sports.

One day in 2011 though, that all changed for me.

I was working a demanding job at the time which involved extended shifts. As a result, my sleep was affected, and I wasn't getting enough sleep each night. I knew this particular project at work was critical though, so I forced myself to get up each day, despite being exhausted and sleep deprived.

After more than a week of this, my boss finally pulled me aside and told me to go see the doctor, because apparently, I looked green! And of course, I felt awful. The doctor did some tests and had me check in to the hospital, where a blood test showed positive for EBV (Epstein-Barr virus, or Mono as its also known.)

The next few days were spent lying in a hospital bed, sleeping 15-20 hours per day, and taking Tylenol-3's for the pain. I have never felt fatigue on that scale before. I was so tired that it physically hurt.

Eventually I was sent home, where I continued sleeping 12–15-hour days for a couple weeks. After about a month, my body required only 8-10 hours of sleep, which was an improvement.

Feeling that this episode was now behind me, I then decided to try some calisthenics and push-ups, since I had not been active for some time. Soon after I started though, I experienced a level of fatigue that approached what I experienced in the hospital. The next three days were spent sleeping roughly 12 or 13 hours each night until I recovered.

Clearly there was a connection between physical exertion, and the fatigue I was experiencing. Luckily for me, in a few months even this condition cleared up and I was able to more or less resume my normal activities, with one caveat. If I started pushing myself too hard or went a couple days without getting a full night's sleep, I would really start to feel worn down. I took this as my cue to just relax, and take some time for myself. But beyond those occasional bouts of tiredness, I could more or less function normally.

I began working out again, playing sports, and living a full life. Again, I thought my issues with fatigue were behind me.

That all changed again in October 2019. My work at the time had arranged for me to take a trip to the Netherlands and Belgium, where I would meet one of our equipment suppliers for a plant tour, as well as some sightseeing. I was looking forward to this trip!

What I was unprepared for was the unrelenting schedule; late nights, and early mornings where we would need to visit manufacturing plants and job sites. I was getting about five hours a sleep each night. By the sixth night of this routine, my body rebelled.

I felt like I had just come out of the hospital again. I was sleeping fourteen hours a day. The fatigue was on a level that someone without CFS just couldn't understand. Even when I did finally wake up, I felt that even a minimal amount of exertion would just push me over the edge again. I deliberately walked at a slow pace, and moved slowly, to avoid exacerbating my condition. Any little exertion seemed to worsen my symptoms.

Once I got back home, I moved back in with my parents for a while to help me recover. But even after weeks of resting, I felt so fragile. I remember one occasion, when someone rang the doorbell, and I started walking briskly so I could get to the door quickly. But even this was too much for my frail body. The next couple days I spent mostly lying on the couch or in bed. Any exertion left me feeling lightheaded and dizzy.

I also noticed that any activity that involved cortisol production, would make me feel exhausted. For example, heightened stress increased my fatigue. So did fasting. I had to always keep some snacks close by in case I started to go hungry. (Fasting, as you may know, tells your adrenal glands to produce cortisol, the stress hormone.) Coffee, and any caffeinated beverage, also interacts with your nervous system and stimulates cortisol production [1].

Even though in time, my symptoms improved somewhat, I knew that something had changed inside my body. I was never going back to that energy level I enjoyed even post-2011. I had to adjust my expectations for myself, for my life, and any goals that I had planned for myself.

If you've been through this process, you can empathize with how difficult this is. It is very hard to accept that now your life is forever changed, due to circumstances beyond your control. To accept your limitations, and to try and do so with poise and humility, is easier said than done.

But this in itself was a learning experience, and a growing one. I have come to experience that our mindset when going through a trial, can make the difference between viewing ourselves as a failure, or seeing it as a steppingstone to eventual success. In Chapter three of this book, I will go into more detail with some of the tools I used to help me over this difficult period.

---

[1] William R. Lovallo, PhD, Thomas L. Whitsett, MD, Mustafa al'Absi, PhD, Bong Hee Sung, PhD, Andrea S. Vincent, PhD, and Michael F. Wilson, MD. Caffeine Stimulation of Cortisol Secretion Across the Waking Hours in Relation to Caffeine Intake Levels; 2008. Retrieved from: https://www.ncbi.nlm.nih.gov/pmc/articles/PMC2257922/

Chapter Two: Understanding Chronic Fatigue Syndrome

Before telling you how I started my journey to recovery, this would be a good time to define what chronic fatigue syndrome is.

The Center for Disease Control and Prevention (CDC) has suggested the following symptoms as a basis for diagnosing CFS:

> "Myalgic encephalomyelitis/chronic fatigue syndrome (ME/CFS) is a serious , long-term illness that affects many body systems. People with ME/CFS are often not able to do their usual activities. At times, ME/CFS may confine them to bed. People with ME/CFS have severe fatigue and sleep problems. ME/CFS may get worse after people with the illness try to do as much as they want or need to do. This symptom is called post-exertional malaise (PEM). Other symptoms can include problems with thinking and concentrating, pain, and dizziness."   (CDC, 2023)

Unfortunately, there is insufficient research as to the causes of CFS, although several studies point to the pre-existence of a viral infection (Epstein-Barr virus or Herpes) as a common precursor to CFS. I'll go into more detail on this later.

No Help From the Establishment

My family doctor requested the standard check-box tests for low energy: Thyroid, Iron, Cortisol. Everything checked out.

My next option was to visit a naturopath. The first naturopath I visited recommended a cleanse to rid my body of parasites. I also changed my diet. I took a 'food sensitivity' test, and reduced or eliminated those foods which were identified as causing an immune reaction. I also switched to a low-inflammation diet, also on the recommendations of the N.D.

Neither of these steps resulted in a substantive improvement of symptoms. So, I kept trying different naturopaths.

Another N.D. suggested I take supplements to support my adrenal glands, such as adaptogens and adrenal gland extract. While I did find these to be situationally helpful, such as when I was more run down than usual, neither of these addressed the underlying causes of my symptoms.

Additionally, I had spent a considerable amount of money on doctors' visits, tests, and expensive supplements. I was beginning to lose hope.

The Missing Link

Around this time, a friend of mine had given me a referral to Dr. Rose Bilotta. Dr. Bilotta is a Public Health and Preventive Medicine Specialist in Canada, who is also an Institute of Functional Medicine Certified Practitioner (IFMCP) and physician nutrition specialist.

Dr. Bilotta pointed out some of the research that had been done in the field of CFS in patients who previously suffered a viral infection. I encourage you to read some of the research yourself; by checking the sources in the footnotes in this Chapter. There are several studies which show a causal link between persistent CFS symptoms and having been diagnosed with certain viral infections in the past.

This includes Mononucleosis, Epstein-Barr virus, and HHV-6 (Human herpesvirus 6) [2]. Studies showed that treatment with the antiviral Valacyclovir reduced symptoms of CFS/ME, as well as antibody titers and cardiac symptoms [3]. In the study conducted by Dr. Henderson, 93% of the adolescent patients treated with valacyclovir had a positive

---

[2] HHV-6 Foundation. CFS patients with ciHHV-6 may benefit from antiviral treatment. Retrieved from: https://hhv-6foundation.org/cihhv-6/cfs-patients-with-cihhv-6-may-benefit-from-antiviral-treatment

[3] Lerner, Martin A. Valacyclovir treatment in Epstein-Barr virus subset chronic fatigue syndrome: thirty-six months follow-up; 2007. Retrieved from: https://pubmed.ncbi.nlm.nih.gov/18019402/.

response! [4] For me, this confirmed my theory that there was a connection with my previous viral infection.

Not all medical practitioners agree over these findings, as some claim that such viruses should show up in a patient's bloodwork, if indeed they are present in the body.

Dr. Theodore Henderson, MD, PhD, explains why this would not be the case:

> "Over the years, my findings have been challenged by physicians performing PCR on the blood of my CFS/ME patients and not finding DNA for any herpes viruses. If a patient has HHV6 in the neurons of their brain, where it is happily replicating and spreading via axonal transport, why would you expect to find HHV6 DNA in the blood? Patients with cold sores rarely have signs of HSV1 DNA in their bloodstream and patients with active herpetic lesions of the genitalia rarely have a detectable serum viral load. Prusty and colleagues [5] examined the blood of patients with confirmed CFS/ME for HHV6 DNA or RNA. Indeed, no more than 40% showed evidence of HHV6 in the blood." [6]

The Role of Mitochondria

Mitochondria are known as the "energy factories" of the body. They provide energy to our cells by means of a chemical known as adenosine triphosphate (ATP).

---

[4] Henderson, TA. Valacyclovir treatment of chronic fatigue in adolescents; 2014. Retrieved from: https://pubmed.ncbi.nlm.nih.gov/24445302/

[5] Schreiner P, Harrer T, Scheibenbogen C, et al. Human Herpesvirus-6 Reactivation, Mitochondrial Fragmentation, and the Coordination of Antiviral and Metabolic Phenotypes in Myalgic Encephalomyelitis/Chronic Fatigue Syndrome Retrieved from: https://journals.aai.org/immunohorizons/article/4/4/201/4109/Human-Herpesvirus-6-Reactivation-Mitochondrial; Immunohorizons. 2020;4(4):201-215.

[6] Henderson, TA. Chronic Fatigue Syndrome, Viruses, and the Innate Immune System, 2020; Retrieved from: https://www.psychiatryadvisor.com/home/topics/general-psychiatry/chronic-fatigue-syndrome-viruses-and-the-innate-immune-system/

HHV-6 and other viruses can lie dormant in our systems for years, surfacing only during certain times, such as prolonged stress. Researchers found that HHV-6 is capable of partially reactivating; that is, only a small number of proteins are formed, rather than the complete virus. Yet, these small number of proteins have a profound impact on the cell.

When this happens, ATP production is impaired, and a pro-inflammatory response is invoked. This was demonstrated when researchers introduced healthy cells next to the cells that were partially reactivated with HHV-6. These cells developed a fragmented mitochondria and a pro-inflammatory state, as though they had experienced HHV-6 reactivation themselves [6].

This explained why, despite taking multiple supplements to support my mitochondrial health, they appeared to be ineffective.

My understanding of the above research is that viruses such as Epstein-Barr Virus and HHV-6 can often leave behind "leftovers", such as random virus proteins, that continue to trigger inflammation and immune response in CFS sufferers.

It is perhaps not a coincidence, that many sufferers of "long Covid", as it is being called, have very similar symptoms to those suffering from CFS. It is my hope that with the increased funding going into research of this illness, that a lasting treatment may be on the horizon.

----

[6]

Chapter Three: Daylight

Finally having a theory as to what was happening in my body and why, was satisfying. Discovering that there was a connection between my CFS symptoms, and my previous viral infection, gave me hope that there would be an effective treatment option.

Building your 'Stack'

What follows in this Chapter is the regimen that allowed me to finally beat this illness and achieve symptom relief. I call this combination of medicine and supplements my CFS 'Stack'. A stack is a term borrowed from the bodybuilding world, and simply refers to a collection of supplements you take on a regular basis.

Feel free to experiment with dosages on these supplements to tailor your recovery. For example, I reduced my intake of Cordyceps mushrooms because I found they gave me too much energy, to the point where my sleep was being affected.

Most of these supplements can be purchased online through Amazon or other retailers. And while there is an initial investment of money to purchase them, I promise you the results will be so worth it!

Valacyclovir

The treatment that my doctor (Dr. Bilotta) suggested, was the antiviral drug Valacyclovir. Again, I am not a medical professional nor claim to be; always speak with your health care professional before starting any medication.

Valacyclovir is an antiviral medication used to treat infections caused by the herpes simplex virus (HSV) and varicella-zoster virus (VZV). Valacyclovir is often used to treat genital herpes, cold sores (oral herpes), and shingles. It works by stopping the virus from replicating and spreading, which can reduce the severity and duration of symptoms, and may also help to prevent future outbreaks.

Valacyclovir is generally well-tolerated, but common side effects can include headache, nausea, and stomach pain. It is important to take valacyclovir exactly as prescribed by a healthcare provider, as the dosage and duration of treatment may vary depending on the specific condition being treated.

Upon beginning my treatment with Valacyclovir, my doctor informed me that if I noticed improvement in my symptoms, that I would need to remain on the drug indefinitely. And indeed, I noticed that if I missed my dose even by a few hours, the feelings of light-headedness and fatigue would return quickly.

I followed my recommended dosage for the first month, after which I tapered to a maintenance dose of 1000mg daily for ongoing support.

Within the first month of starting Valacyclovir, I felt a dramatic improvement in my symptoms. It was like night and day. Clearly, this drug was the missing link I had been looking for.

I felt "normal" for the first time in a long time! I gradually began re-introducing light exercise into my daily routine and becoming more active.

I was so excited in fact, that I foolishly decided to go back to the gym and resume my intense weightlifting routine that I loved. However, my body was not ready for this, and I suffered another relapse of fatigue. So I would caution you, please learn from my mistake. It is better to introduce a *gradual* program of light to moderate exercise into your routine. Only increase the intensity once you can comfortably handle that level of exertion. I will go into more detail on graded exercise later in this book.

The introduction of Valacyclovir was the most crucial ingredient to my gradual recovery. But it was not the only one.

While Valacyclovir got me most of the way there, I discovered a few supplements that really helped support my energy level and round out my recovery. Some of these supplements I take daily, others situationally.

Keep in mind that what worked for me, may not work for you. Always consult your health care provider before taking any supplements, especially if you are currently taking any medication or have an underlying health condition.

My Experience with CCNM

I feel very fortunate that I was able to come across the Canadian College of Naturopathic Medicine. As I mentioned in the beginning of the book, I had visited naturopaths before. I'm not trying to knock them; they can be very beneficial depending on what your condition is.

What I really liked about the approach of CCNM, was that you are dealing with a team of doctors and students. In my appointments, I met with two grad students, who were working under the supervision of a registered naturopathic doctor. These guys were eager, and enthusiastic in their desire to not only help me with my condition, but to really investigate and try to figure out what was going on. I can't recommend them enough.

After several weeks of trial-and-error, my team found two supplements that were of great help to my condition.

Rhodiola

Rhodiola rosea is a herb that grows in cold, mountainous regions of Europe and Asia. It has been used for centuries as a natural remedy for various health conditions, especially those related to stress and fatigue. Rhodiola is considered an adaptogen, which means it helps the body adapt to different kinds of stress and maintain balance.

As an adaptogen, rhodiola may help restore the body's resilience to stress, thus preventing or reducing the effects of chronic stress on the body and mind. Rhodiola may also help improve energy levels, mental clarity, mood stability, sleep quality, and overall well-being by modulating the hormones, neurotransmitters, antioxidants, and blood flow in the body.

Several studies have shown that rhodiola can effectively reduce fatigue and improve quality of life in people with chronic fatigue syndrome (CFS), burnout syndrome (BS), or other stress-related disorders. For example:

- In a randomized controlled trial involving 100 people with CFS symptoms, rhodiola extract (400 mg per day for 8 weeks) significantly improved stress symptoms, fatigue levels, quality of life scores, mood scores, and concentration scores compared to placebo. [7]

- In a systematic review of 11 randomized controlled trials involving 714 participants with various stress-related conditions, rhodiola extract (50–680 mg per day for 2–12 weeks) significantly improved physical and mental fatigue, depression, anxiety, and quality of life compared to placebo or control interventions. [8]

---

[7]Yevgeniya Lekomtseva, Irina Zhukova, Anna Wacker. Rhodiola rosea in Subjects with Prolonged or Chronic Fatigue Symptoms: Results of an Open-Label Clinical Trial ; 2017. Retrieved from: https://pubmed.ncbi.nlm.nih.gov/28219059/

[8]Jay D Amsterdam, Alexander G Panossian. Rhodiola rosea L. as a putative botanical antidepressant, 2016. Retrieved from: https://pubmed.ncbi.nlm.nih.gov/27013349/

* * *

These studies suggest that rhodiola may be a safe and effective natural remedy for chronic fatigue and its associated symptoms. However, more research is needed to confirm its long-term efficacy and safety, as well as to determine the optimal dosage, duration, and method of administration for different individuals and conditions.

Another way that rhodiola can help improve energy is by enhancing the function of the mitochondria, the energy-producing structures in cells. Rhodiola has been shown to have antioxidant effects, which can help protect the mitochondria from damage and increase their energy-producing ability.

In chapter two, I provide several references showing how mitochondrial function in CFS patients is impaired. I believe that, used in conjunction with Valacyclovir, it offers powerful support to the mitochondria.

I noticed a definite improvement once I started taking rhodiola. My jogging sessions would last much longer, and I did not feel so fatigued afterward, so this supplement is one I continue to take regularly.

While I supplemented with rhodiola daily, my team at CCNM suggested that this herb should not be taken on a continual basis, but to cycle off it occasionally, to avoid building a tolerance. For example, I would take the supplement daily for one month, then cycle off it for one to two weeks.

D-Ribose

D-Ribose is a type of sugar that is naturally produced by the body from glucose. It is an essential component of ATP, which is the molecule that stores and releases energy in the cells. D-Ribose also helps build RNA, which is the genetic material that carries instructions for protein synthesis.

D-Ribose: The Research

The idea behind using D-ribose for PEM is that by increasing the production of ATP, it may help improve energy levels and reduce feelings of fatigue.

Some people with chronic fatigue syndrome (CFS) or fibromyalgia (FM) may have low levels of ATP in their muscles and nerves, which can cause symptoms such as fatigue, pain, poor sleep, and cognitive impairment. D-Ribose supplements may help increase ATP production and improve these symptoms.

Several studies have shown that D-Ribose can significantly improve energy, well-being, sleep quality, mental clarity, and pain intensity in people with CFS or FM. For example, a pilot study published in The Journal of Alternative and Complementary Medicine found that taking 5 grams of D-Ribose three times a day for three weeks resulted in an average 61.3% increase in energy, 37% increase in overall well-being, 29.3% improvement in sleep, 30% improvement in mental clarity, and 15.6% decrease in pain. A larger multicenter trial confirmed these findings.

Other research has indicated that supplementing with D-ribose may help improve energy levels, reduce muscle soreness, and increase physical performance in people with CFS. One small study of 41 patients showed that D-ribose was well-tolerated, and resulted in a significant improvement in energy, sleep, mental clarity, pain, and well-being. [9] The majority of the patients (66%) reported an average increase in energy of 45%.

Ribose: Additional Health Benefits

Some of the additional benefits of D-ribose supplementation are:

---

[9] Jacob E Teitelbaum, Clarence Johnson, John St Cyr. *"The use of D-ribose in chronic fatigue syndrome and fibromyalgia: a pilot study"*. Retrieved from: https://pubmed.ncbi.nlm.nih.gov/17109576

• It helps restore energy levels in your cells after intense exercise or stress. Some studies have shown that D-ribose supplements can increase ATP levels in muscle cells after strenuous activity, which may reduce muscle soreness and fatigue .

• It can improve heart function and blood flow in people with coronary artery disease or congestive heart failure. D-ribose supplements may enhance the ability of the heart to pump blood and oxygen to the tissues, which may improve symptoms and quality of life .

• It may reduce pain and fatigue in people with chronic fatigue syndrome or fibromyalgia. These conditions are characterized by low levels of ATP and impaired energy metabolism in the cells. D-ribose supplements may help increase ATP production and reduce oxidative stress, which may alleviate some of the symptoms .

Dosage and Usage

D-Ribose is generally well tolerated and has few side effects. However, it may lower blood sugar levels, so people with diabetes or hypoglycemia should consult their doctor before taking it. D-Ribose may also interact with some medications, such as anticoagulants or antiplatelets. Therefore, it is important to talk to your healthcare provider before starting any supplement.

D-Ribose is available as a powder or capsule form in health food stores and online. The recommended dosage is 5 grams three times a day for three weeks, followed by a maintenance dose of 5 grams twice a day as needed. You can mix the powder with water or juice, or take it with food.

If you have CFS or FM and are looking for a natural way to boost your energy and reduce your symptoms, D-Ribose may be worth a try. However, remember that supplements are not regulated by the FDA and may vary in quality and purity. Always choose a reputable brand that has been tested by a third-party organization, such as USP,

ConsumerLab, or NSF. And don't forget to inform your doctor about any supplements you are taking or planning to take.

Consult your health care provider on the dosage you should be taking for Ribose. While this is a supplement you can take daily, you can choose to only take it before physical activity, if you want to reduce the amount of pills and powders you take every day. This supplement is particularly helpful when taken before and after exercise.

Before playing sports for example, I would always remember to take my Ribose supplement. When I didn't, I would need to rest the next day and not do any physical activity. But my energy level was much better if I took my Ribose supplement before and after exercise.

In summary, Ribose is a great addition to anyone suffering from CFS/ME or Post Exertional Malaise (PEM), and is backed up not only by the study mentioned above, but many anecdotal reports as well.

Graded Exercise

Graded exercise was another adjustment to my lifestyle that was recommended by my team at CCNM. A graded exercise program can be an effective way to increase energy levels for people with chronic fatigue syndrome (CFS). Here's how it works. A graded exercise program involves gradually increasing physical activity over time. This is because people with CFS often experience a worsening of symptoms after physical exertion, which can make them reluctant to engage in physical activity. By starting with a low level of activity and gradually increasing it, people with CFS can build up their tolerance for exercise and avoid exacerbating their symptoms.

The program should be customized to meet the individual needs of each person with CFS. This means that the program is tailored to their current level of physical fitness, their specific symptoms, and their goals for increasing energy levels.

If you happen to live near a public pool or aquatic center, swimming laps is a great activity, since it is not a high-impact activity, and you can modulate your exertion as much as you like. Try gradually increasing not only the number of laps you complete, but your pace as well. After a few weeks, I could comfortably swim nearly twenty minutes continuously.

A graded exercise program may include a combination of aerobic exercise, such as walking, cycling, or swimming, and strength training, such as resistance band exercises or weightlifting. This combination of activities can help to increase energy levels by improving cardiovascular function and building muscle strength.

The key to success with graded exercise is to closely monitor your progress, and be patient. If you increase your activity too much, too quickly, you may exacerbate your symptoms and suffer a crash. If your symptoms worsen upon starting, the exercise program may be adjusted accordingly.

Regular exercise has been shown to have a positive impact on mental health, which can also help to increase energy levels for people with CFS. Exercise can help to reduce stress, improve mood, and boost self-esteem, which can help to increase energy levels and overall well-being.

My personal program started off with only walking. My initial goal was to complete a total of half a kilometer every day for one week, then increasing to one kilometer the following week. After I felt comfortable with that, I would keep increasing it gradually. Eventually, I began to incorporate periods of light jogging with my walk, and increasing those periods each time until I could jog comfortably for several minutes at a time. Soon I was able to comfortably jog or cycle for twenty to thirty minutes at a time.

A graded exercise program can be an effective way to increase energy levels for people with CFS. By gradually increasing physical activity, customizing the program to meet individual needs, and monitoring progress, people with CFS can safely build their endurance and improve their overall health and well-being. However, it's important to consult with a doctor or a physical therapist before starting any new exercise program, especially if you have any underlying medical conditions.

Further Research

There is a very helpful Facebook group called "Chronic Fatigue Sydrome Support Group" which is free to join. Every once in a while, you'll get different members sharing tips on what helped them manage their CFS symptoms. After talking with these members one-on-one, I decided to do my own research, as well as try these supplements for myself.

The supplements listed below are the result of this research as well as trying these supplements for myself. These supplements are what pushed my recovery to a level where Chronic Fatigue is not something that I needed to think about on a regular basis.

NADH/NMN and Coenzyme Q10

NADH (Nicotinamide Adenine Dinucleotide) and NMN (Nicotinamide Mononucleotide) are both important molecules involved in cellular energy metabolism and the regulation of various biological processes. While they are related to each other, they have distinct roles and functions within the body.

NADH is a coenzyme that plays a crucial role in the production of adenosine triphosphate (ATP), which is the main energy currency of cells. It is involved in redox reactions, acting as an electron carrier, and is particularly important in the process of oxidative phosphorylation, which occurs in the mitochondria. NADH is derived from the B-vitamin niacin (also known as vitamin B3).

On the other hand, NMN is a precursor to NAD+ (Nicotinamide Adenine Dinucleotide), which is the oxidized form of NADH. NMN is converted into NAD+ through a series of enzymatic reactions in the body.

There are several studies that you can find online, which show a marked improvement in ME/CFS symptoms when supplementing with NADH/NMN.

The study referenced in this book showed promising results when NADH was combined with Coenzyme Q10 [10].

Coenzyme Q10 (CoQ10) is a naturally occurring compound found in every cell of the body. It plays a crucial role in the production of adenosine triphosphate (ATP), which is the main source of energy for cellular processes.

As you have no doubt deduced by the function of these two supplements, they both assist your body in forming the essential molecule ATP, which is the fuel for our cells. While healthy people do not need this additional fuel, the partial impairment of mitochondria in CFS sufferers may be responsible for the increased demand for this molecule.

In talking with my colleagues in the CFS Support Group on Facebook, the consensus was that the dosage needed to be high; close to 1000mg daily. This is the dose that I took, and which worked for me. I noticed a huge improvement upon starting supplementation with NMN.

NMN powder can be expensive, especially if you're buying it in capsule form. I recommend buying it in bulk instead. On my website, endchronicfatigue.org, I have a link posted to a supplier that sells NMN in powder form.

---

[10] Jesús Castro-Marrero, Maria Jose Segundo, Marcos Lacasa, Alba Martinez-Martinez, Ramon Sanmartin Sentañes, Jose Alegre-Martin: Effect of Dietary Coenzyme Q10 Plus NADH Supplementation on Fatigue Perception and Health-Related Quality of Life in Individuals with Myalgic Encephalomyelitis/Chronic Fatigue Syndrome: A Prospective, Randomized, Double-Blind, Placebo-Controlled Trial; Retrieved from: https://pubmed.ncbi.nlm.nih.gov/34444817/

Olive Leaf Extract

Olive leaf extract is derived from the leaves of the olive tree (Olea europaea). It has been traditionally used for its potential health benefits, including its antiviral properties. However, it's important to note that scientific research on the specific effects of olive leaf extract on viruses is still limited, and more studies are needed to establish its effectiveness in this regard.

That being said, some preliminary research and laboratory studies suggest that olive leaf extract may have antiviral activity against certain viruses. It is believed that the active compounds in olive leaf extract, such as oleuropein and hydroxytyrosol, may help inhibit the replication of viruses and reduce their ability to infect cells. These compounds have been shown to have antimicrobial and immune-stimulating properties.

Olive leaf extract has been studied for its potential effects against various viruses, including herpes viruses, influenza viruses, and respiratory syncytial virus (RSV). Some studies have indicated that it may help inhibit the growth of these viruses in laboratory settings. However, it's important to recognize that these results are from 'in vitro' studies, not from live human testing.

In "Prescription for Herbal Healing" written by Phyllis A. Balch, CNC states:

"Physicians have reported that folks with chronic fatigue and fibromyalgia are often helped by olive leaf extract. People with these syndromes have reported recovery within one month of taking the supplement. They need reported higher spirits, more energy, and a stronger sense of well-being." [11]

The theory is that this supplement assists the body in lowering the total viral load, similar to the way Valacyclovir functions. In fact, I found

---

[11] Balch, Phyllis A. Prescription for Herbal Healing. Penguin Group (USA), 2012

these two remedies to complement each other, and the addition of Olive Leaf Extract marked a definite improvement in my symptoms.

• • •

Cordyceps Mushrooms

Cordyceps mushrooms have been traditionally used in traditional Chinese medicine for centuries and have gained popularity as a potential treatment for various health conditions, including chronic fatigue.

There are several mechanisms by which this supplement benefits those suffering from fatigue issues.

Adaptogenic properties: Cordyceps mushrooms are considered adaptogens, which means they may help the body adapt to stress and normalize its functions. Chronic fatigue is often associated with increased stress and imbalances in the body. Cordyceps mushrooms may help regulate the body's response to stress, potentially reducing fatigue.

Energy production: Cordyceps mushrooms contain bioactive compounds that are believed to enhance energy production and utilization in the body. These compounds, such as cordycepin and adenosine, have been suggested to improve cellular energy production and mitochondrial function, which may contribute to reducing fatigue.

Immune modulation: Chronic fatigue is sometimes associated with immune dysregulation. Cordyceps mushrooms have been found to possess immunomodulatory properties, which means they can help regulate the immune system's response. By supporting immune balance, cordyceps mushrooms may indirectly alleviate fatigue symptoms associated with immune dysfunction.

Oxygen utilization and circulation: Cordyceps mushrooms have been traditionally used to support lung and respiratory function. Improved oxygen utilization and circulation may enhance energy levels and alleviate fatigue.

Anti-inflammatory effects: Chronic fatigue can be associated with systemic inflammation. Cordyceps mushrooms contain compounds that possess anti-inflammatory properties, which may help reduce inflammation in the body and subsequently improve fatigue symptoms.

Cordyceps mushrooms is (kind of) the final supplement I've added to my daily regimen. The Valacyclovir is what got me 70% of the way to recovery, and these additional supplements brought me the rest of the way.

It may seem like a lot to keep track of, as there are six different supplements regularly. But I find that with a little organization early in the week, as well as a pill organizer which I keep on my dresser, after a while it will just become part of your morning routine. And once you begin to experience the benefits of increased energy and productivity, you will no doubt view the inconvenience of taking supplements as a small price to pay for an improved quality of life.

If you need even more of an energy boost, read on for my final supplement recommendation.

PQQ (Pyrroloquinoline Quinone)

Before explaining what this supplement does, I want to point out that adding PQQ to your daily 'stack' is optional. The previous supplements listed here should get you to a full recovery. But if you anticipate a higher than normal level of stress or physical activity coming up, adding PQQ, at least temporarily, will definitely help. PQQ is great for that extra boost of energy. And you'll see why as I explain what it does.

PQQ is a natural compound that is found in some plant foods, such as kiwi, parsley, green peppers, and green tea. PQQ is also produced by some bacteria in your gut. PQQ has many health benefits, but one of its most remarkable effects is on your mitochondria.

Mitochondria are the tiny organelles that produce energy in your cells. They are often called the "powerhouses" of the cell, because they generate ATP, the molecule that fuels all your biological processes. Mitochondria are essential for your health and vitality, but they can also become damaged or dysfunctional due to aging, stress, toxins, infections, and other factors. When your mitochondria are impaired, your energy production declines, and you may experience symptoms such as fatigue, muscle weakness, pain, cognitive impairment, and mood disorders.

PQQ can help restore your mitochondrial function in several ways. First, PQQ can protect your existing mitochondria from oxidative stress and inflammation, which are two major causes of mitochondrial damage. PQQ is a powerful antioxidant that can scavenge free radicals and reduce inflammation in your cells. PQQ can also modulate the expression of genes that are involved in mitochondrial function and protection.

Second, PQQ can stimulate the growth of new mitochondria in your cells. This process is called mitochondrial biogenesis, and it is crucial for maintaining optimal energy levels and cellular health. PQQ can activate a protein called PGC-1alpha, which is the master regulator of mitochondrial biogenesis. PGC-1alpha can trigger the production of more mitochondria in your cells, as well as enhance their efficiency and resilience.

By protecting and enhancing your mitochondria, PQQ can help you combat chronic fatigue and ME. Several studies have shown that PQQ supplementation can improve energy levels, physical performance, cognitive function, sleep quality, and mood in healthy adults and elderly people. PQQ may also have specific benefits for people with chronic fatigue and ME, who often have impaired mitochondrial function and reduced energy production.

For example, one study found that PQQ supplementation improved fatigue scores and reduced oxidative stress in patients with fibromyalgia (FM), a condition that is closely related to chronic fatigue syndrome (CFS) or ME. Another study found that PQQ supplementation increased blood flow to the cerebral cortex, which is the part of the brain that is responsible for attention, thinking, and memory. This may help improve cognitive function and reduce brain fog in people with chronic fatigue and ME.

PQQ is generally safe and well-tolerated, with no serious side effects reported. The optimal dosage of PQQ for chronic fatigue and ME is not established yet, but most studies have used doses ranging from 10 to 20 mg per day. You may want to start with a lower dose and gradually increase it until you notice positive effects. You may also want to combine PQQ with other supplements that support mitochondrial function, such as CoQ10, D-ribose, calcium pyruvate, and resveratrol. My usual dosage is 20 mg daily, and I take a supplement that includes CoQ10 as well.

PQQ is a promising supplement for chronic fatigue and ME sufferers who want to boost their energy levels and improve their quality of life. By protecting and enhancing your mitochondria, PQQ can help you overcome the symptoms of fatigue, weakness, pain, cognitive impairment, and mood disorders. If you are interested in trying PQQ for yourself, consult with your doctor first and look for a reputable brand that provides high-quality PQQ products.

Chapter Four: The Power of Perspective

Managing an illness involves so much more than supplements and exercise. That is why I consider this chapter just as essential as the previous ones. CFS is something that is very likely going to accompany us for the rest of our lives. As mentioned earlier, you will experience setbacks on the road to success. So learning to live with this illness, and adjusting our attitude towards it, will make the difference between surviving, and thriving.

Dealing with a   Relapse

The steps I've described in the previous Chapter have helped me to almost eliminate this illness and have a normal life again. Despite this, I do not claim to have found a 'cure', but rather, an effective way of managing it.

This means that you will have setbacks. It could be from exercising too hard, pushing yourself too hard at work or in social events, or just an extended period of poor sleep. When these happen, and they will, it's important not to forget the tremendous progress you've already made!

It's a lot like climbing a flight of stairs. Just because you trip and stumble a few steps, doesn't mean you have to start from the very bottom! Just pick yourself up and keep on climbing. Setbacks can be viewed as steppingstones on the long journey to success and living the life you want.

Obstacle or Opportunity?

Learning that you have a chronic illness can feel a lot like losing a loved one in death. Thus, its healthy and important to allow yourself time to grieve this loss. In fact, you may have lost more than just your health; your job, and your independence can also have been affected.

Dr. Kitty Stein, who herself has multiple sclerosis, says: "You've got to mourn what's lost, but you also need to understand what's still there." [12]

A sailor cannot control a storm, but they can adjust his response to it, by adjusting their sails and bearing. You may not be able to control the 'storm' of this illness, but you can adjust your sails, so to speak, by adjusting your physical, mental, and emotional resources to cope with this change.

You Are not Powerless

In his bestselling book *The Obstacle Is the Way*, Ryan Holiday tells the story of Rubin "Hurricane" Carter, a top contender for the middleweight title in the 1960s. At the height of his career, he was falsely accused of a crime he did not commit: triple homicide. At his bogus trial, he received a biased verdict of life imprisonment. It was a terrible fate for someone who was on the verge of fame and success. I will quote from the book what happens next:

> "Carter reported to prison in an expensive, tailored suit, wearing a $5,000 diamond ring and a gold watch. And so, waiting in line to be entered into the general inmate population, he asked to speak to someone in charge.

> "Looking the warden in the eye, Carter proceeded to inform him and the guards that he was not giving up the last thing he controlled: himself. In his remarkable declaration, he told them, in so many words, 'I know you had nothing to do with the

---

[12] Qtd. in "Living Successfully With Your Ailment – How?" -jw.org

injustice that brought me to this jail, so I'm willing to stay here until I get out. But I will not, under any circumstances, be treated like a prisoner—because I am not and never will be   *powerless* .'"[13]

Carter refused to despair, wear a uniform, attend parole hearings, or try to get his sentence reduced. Instead, he devoted every waking hour to his case. He would read books on law, philosophy, and history. He was determined to appeal and win his case, and he would devote all his time and energies in prison towards that goal. He would leave prison not only a free man, but a better one.

After nineteen long years, and two trials, the verdict was finally overturned, and Carter could leave prison as a free man. He did not seek damages or request an apology. Because to Carter, that would imply that he was powerless, and that they'd taken something from him. Instead, he was the one who decided how the experience would affect him.

Nelson Mandela, the anti-apartheid leader who was jailed 27 years for his activism, and later became the president of South Africa, drew inspiration from the poem   *Invictus* during his imprisonment. It reads:

> Out of the night that covers me,
>   Black as the pit from pole to pole,
> I thank whatever gods may be
>   For my unconquerable soul.
>
> In the fell clutch of circumstance
>   I have not winced nor cried aloud.
> Under the bludgeonings of chance
>   My head is bloody, but unbowed.
>
> Beyond this place of wrath and tears
>   Looms but the Horror of the shade,

---

[13] Holiday, Ryan. The Obstacle Is the Way. London, England. Profile Books, 2015

And yet the menace of the years
  Finds and shall find me unafraid.

It matters not how strait the gate,
  How charged with punishments the scroll,
I am the master of my fate,
  I am the captain of my soul.

–"Invictus", by William Ernest Henley

How we *perceive* our situation is up to us. No one can make us feel defeated or give up hope; only we can do that. We can't always choose our circumstances in life, but we can choose how we respond to them. We gain tremendous power once we realize that we are not the victims of our circumstances.

Set Attainable Goals

In prison, Carter realized he still had his mind, lots of time, and ability to plan and act. He spent his time accordingly.

Because of our illness, there may be things we can no longer do. Instead of dwelling on what was lost, focus your energy on what you still *can* do. What attributes and abilities do you have right now, that you can use to improve your situation? Can you learn a new skill? Reconnect with an old friend? Help someone in need? Helping others helps us put our problems in perspective. There is always someone worse off than we are.

Goals help direct our mind towards the future. They give us a sense of accomplishment and can also restore our self-confidence.

In his 2014 commencement address to the University of Texas (and in his bestselling book "Make Your Bed"), Admiral William McRaven, US Navy SEAL, explains why the simple act of making his bed every morning was so important:

• • •

"It was a simple task, mundane at best. But every morning, we were required to make our bed to perfection. But the wisdom of this simple act has been proven to me, many times over. If you make your bed every morning, you will have accomplished the first task of the day. It will give you a small sense of pride, and will encourage you to do another task. And another, and another. And at the end of the day, that one task completed, will have turned into many tasks completed. Making your bed will also reinforce the fact that the little things in life matter. If you can't do the little things right, you'll never be able to do the big things right. And if by chance you have a miserable day, you will come home to a bed that is made – that you have made – and a made bed gives you the encouragement that tomorrow will be better." (YouTube, 2014) [14]

The simple act of completing a task, however small, can give us the motivation we need to continue setting goals and moving forward.

---

[14] The University of Texas at Austin. "Admiral McRaven addresses the University of Texas at Austin Class of 2014". YouTube, uploaded by The University of Texas at Austin, 2014, https://www.youtube.com/watch?v=yaQZFhrWofU

• • •

The Path Ahead

My personal experience in using the methods described in this book, has resulted in a significant improvement in my symptoms. In 2011, I never thought I'd be able to play beach volleyball with my friends, or have a late night out of socializing, and to be fine the next day. Of course, I still need to be careful about over-extending myself or going too long without enough sleep. My energy level is still something I need to be aware of and manage.

For those days when you just need to rest, it's helpful having some hobbies that can help you pass the time. View it as an opportunity to do some reading, play video games, or call up some friends you haven't spoken to in a while. Try to do a little bit each day to move you closer to your goals.

I decided to start an online course in Web Development. It might not ever turn into anything more than a hobby, but I am learning a new skill and it reminds me that I can set meaningful goals and reach them.

Sometimes we deal with multiple issues in our life at once. And if those times happen to coincide with an episode of excessive fatigue, it can be unusually hard to deal with.

At those times, remember that this condition is temporary. Things will get better. Sometimes we can get so focused on our problems and what we can't do that we develop tunnel vision. We become fixated on what we've lost, and we lose sight of what's still in front of us. Talk to a friend who has endured adversity and learn from them. Take some extra time for yourself. You may not be able to run a marathon, but you can go for a walk outside. Walking, especially in nature, has a calming effect and can reduce our anxiety. Nature reconnects us with the larger world and helps us put our problems in perspective. And walking a predetermined number of steps is an achievable goal that can give you a sense of accomplishment. I have been on many long walks when that was one of the few activities I could actually do.

As mentioned in Chapter four, the down time you will experience because of this illness can be a great opportunity to learn a new skill. At the very least, we can view it as an opportunity to build *resilience*. I certainly haven't mastered this quality, but I'm convinced that it's one we can learn, and I'm trying to learn and apply it more each day.

I truly hope that my experience will provide some hope for those who are suffering from this illness. There is hope for you. This illness is a detour, not a death sentence.

About the Author

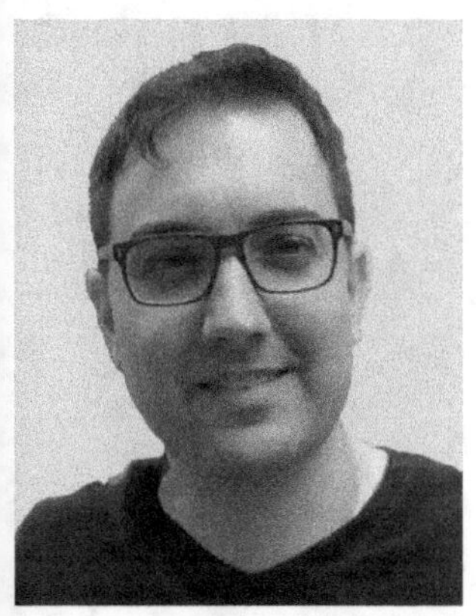

Andre Di Carlo lives in Toronto, Canada. He has a passion for sport, particularly soccer and cycling. 'How I Beat my Chronic Fatigue Syndrome' is his first self-published book.